FINDING PURPOSE AND MEANING

Sally Survives Her Brief, Nasty Dance with Psychiatry

ALEXANDER T. POLGAR PH. D.

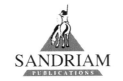

Sandriam Publication

Hamilton, Ontario, Canada

FINDING PURPOSE AND MEANING:
SALLY SURVIVES HER BRIEF, NASTY DANCE WITH PSYCHIATRY

© 2020 Sandriam Publications Inc.
183 St. Clair Blvd.
Hamilton, Ontario, Canada
L8M 2N9

atpolgar@sympatico.ca
www.atpolgar.com/sandriam-publications

ISBN: 978-1-9990954-8-2

Printed and bound in Canada

Cover: Workhorse Design Studio

ALSO BY ALEXANDER T. POLGAR, PH.D.

Conducting Parenting Capacity Assessments: A Manual for Mental Health Professionals

Chronobiology: Strategies for Coping with Shift Work

Because We Can – We Must: Achieving the Human Developmental Potential in Five Generations

TWO: One Destined to Addiction the Other to be Free

Freedom: Sally Gets Sober and Starts to Grow Up

For Janis

Contents

I FOUND PURPOSE AND MEANING BECAUSE I SURVIVED MY BRIEF, NASTY DANCE WITH PSYCHIATRY

I am Sally, and this third book of four in my trilogy, like the previous two, is not a thriller. I will not take you on a long and twisted road with many bumps and turns and then surprise you with an ending you would never have guessed. I will, however, frighten you several times along the way, probably make many of you angry, even furious but mostly I hope to make you glad to know information which might just save your life or the life of someone you love.

This third book, in fact, was inspired by someone I met on my journey who could have used the information, herself. Unfortunately, I did not know then what I know now and, as a result, could not help her. For no other reason than being the kind of person I am, stubbornly curious, I survived a very dangerous time on my journey to sustained abstinence. Mary was not as fortunate, and she died. The 'treatments' which took her life were well-intentioned, perhaps even the best in the field of psychiatry; nevertheless, she died. Like me, all Mary wanted was some relief from the lousy feelings she was not familiar with because before she had them, most of the time, she was stoned, drunk or both. For her innocent, naïve and trusting ask for help, she died.

I am driven, therefore, to write this third story in part out of survival- guilt and, in part, to help prevent others from becoming another fatality, like Mary.

Someone told me that to get your point across, it must be repeated several times. I also heard that it is a good idea to say it in different ways, and that you should repeat yourself at least seven times. Well, I don't know just how many times I repeated myself in the first two books of four in this trilogy, and I sure don't know how many times I will repeat myself in this one. But I do not care if some of you get pissed at me for repeating myself. The message in the books is too important to worry about offending a few impatient, overly-critical people.

I already touched upon the topic of this book in the previous two. In this one, I really want to get into how dangerous it can be to dance with psychiatry. I hope reading this will make you as curious as I was about understanding what bothers you emotionally, why your thinking can become really bizarre, and what makes you behave so badly. Also, I hope reading this will make you think not twice, but several times and ask many questions before you start dancing with some professional claiming to have the ability to 'help' you with prescription drugs.

In the first chapter, I write about the negative emotions that come to the surface, some say to our level of consciousness when we stop drowning them in alcohol and/or drugs. This can be a very dangerous time and it threatens the new and fragile abstinence from all intoxicants for even the most stubborn amongst us.

In the second chapter, I discuss the enormous benefits of a very familiar saying, "If it seems to be too good to be true, it is". I discovered the hard way that there are no easy fixes, and naïve, wishful thinking doesn't make what you want just happen. Also, I describe the dangers of placing unconditional trust in a stranger, regardless of that person's importance or credentials. Trust must be earned, so I learned the hard way.

Ignorance is not bliss when it comes to your mental and physical well being, is the theme of chapter three. You need to ask a lot of questions because, if you don't, bad things could and will happen. In this chapter, some of the horrible side effects of psychiatric drugs are described. This chapter is particularly scary.

In the fourth chapter, the theme of asking questions is repeated and elaborated. When we do not ask important questions, especially of a person about to prescribe a psychiatric drug , horrible, unexpected things can, and do, happen. In this chapter, I also touch upon how the promise of a quick, easy fix and those making it, became so popular. After all, who wants to take responsibility for messing up another person's life? I think very few, which explains the popularity of illness and disease applied to bad behaviour, mental and emotional problems

The fifth chapter is all about experimenting with drugs. It should be a familiar activity, especially for all those recently enjoying a clear mind that comes with abstinence for a few months. As I was writing it, I kept asking myself: "How could you have been so stupid?" But stupid I was, for sure. Not the IQ type, since I'm pretty smart, but the naïve, trusting type, which I hardly ever am. While using, I never put my life at such risk as I did "under the care of the establishment-honoured psychiatrist". But until I came to my senses, I willingly, without question, took this and that prescribed psychiatric drug, replaced this with that and danced with some combinations, until my body said: "That is enough," and dragged my naïve, drugged-up mind back into reality.

The fifth chapter was very painful and difficult to write. I suspect it will be as painful and difficult to read for many of you, especially those who have lost a loved one to similar circumstances. The reason is that in this chapter, I tell the story of Mary whose life was pretty similar to mine. We went our own separate ways when my body and mind had had enough of the psychiatrist-prescribed, so-called medicine, and Mary's falling victim to them. It could have been me, and I know it has been for many of your loved ones. I don't know how this genie, otherwise known as biological psychiatry, can ever be stuffed back into the bottle. At the very least, I hope that after reading this chapter you will think long and hard before you rub that deceptive, and in reality, very dangerous, bottle. Simply, when invited to dance, just say NO!

In the sixth chapter, my aim is to share what I learned the hard way about "mental health" and the players who work in this very important but strange field. Some, so I learned, believe that 'crazy' behaviour is caused by biological things like genes or chemical imbalances. Others believe that the cause is environmental. This latter group says, even if a gene for bad behaviour is ever found, which is highly unlikely, that gene still has to be activated by conditions in one's environment. The point I want to make in this chapter, is that at one time or another, because of life experiences, we could all benefit from some counselling. The challenge is to find the right person. The right person is defined as one you get along with and has a belief that is similar to yours. Namely, that you, in interaction with your environment, create your own problems, not some mythical 'chemical imbalance' or gene that has yet to be found.

In chapters seven and eight, I share (show off) what I learned just by curiously looking things up. Chapter seven is like a term paper for a university, introductory course on the evolution of psychiatry and its silent partner, the psycho-pharmaceutical industry (companies that make drugs for psychiatrists). In this chapter, I share what I learned about what each group of drugs is supposed to do and what they actually do to our minds and bodies. The chapter is not about blaming anyone or any organization; it is about helping you understand whom you are dealing with and what is their primary way of helping you – prescription drugs. The reality is that there are no easy, quick fixes, and chasing one can get you into a whole mess of trouble; some trouble from which you cannot recover, and some that just might even kill you.

The eighth chapter is like a school assignment about the dangers of buying into the establishment-supported myth that mental, emotional and behavioural problems have nothing to do with the harm created by the environments in which we live and raise our children. Instead, the establishment and one of its key players, psychiatry, would have us believe the problems are caused by some medical condition not of our own making. Since it's a medical problem, physicians (psychiatrists) are the best equipped to 'treat' them. Then, I get into what it means to be 'treated' by psychiatric drugs, how these drugs are developed and approved to be prescribed to the likes of us. My intention is to first scare you and then to open your eyes, because when you agree to dance with a psychiatrist, you should do so with eyes as wide open as possible.

The ninth and last chapter in this book is about the importance of getting and staying real. I talk about solving what's causing our mental, emotional, and behavioural problems, not just about focusing on getting relief from them. After all, that is what we were doing when we were using. Why would we continue doing the same thing but with prescription drugs? Exchanging illegal intoxicants for legal ones is no answer and, in fact, can be a very dangerous strategy. Being "real" in this chapter, therefore, is defined as accepting that there is no cure for who we are but, if we understand our demons, with the help of a competent counsellor, we can learn to control them as I learned to control being an addict by regularly attending AA meetings.

Just a quick heads up about my use of words. I consider straight, sober, and abstinent to mean the same thing, i.e. not using anything to alter your state of mind or for that matter also your body.

My alter ego, Dr. Polgar, concludes this book with his reflections. As is his habit, he can get a little too professorial. He tries not to so give him a chance and read his take on my experiences. Most importantly, he gives very important references that I used to get informed about the dangers of dancing with psychiatry. I urge you to read at least one of the references, all of them ideally, just to satisfy your curiosity about what's outside of the box everyone is so eager to keep us in.

CHAPTER 1
No One Warned Me

Being sober long enough for my body to get rid of all the shit I was putting into it produced an unexpected, very unpleasant result no one warned me about. It was as if a huge wave of negativity washed over me and knocked me over. At first, it was nothing specific. I couldn't say I was panicky, anxious, sad or afraid; I just felt lousy. I never felt like that, ever. Much later, I figured out that when using, I never allowed myself to feel so bad. Before, even a hint of feeling badly I quickly shut down. It was easy to do. All I had to do was drink more or do more drugs or do both. When I was a kid, I avoided negative feelings by doing dangerously bad things. That was when I was labelled ADHD. I won't even define again what that stands for. This was the time that I was first given so-called medicine. You might recall from the first book, TWO, how well I tolerated that poison. No matter, the point I want to make is that I never let myself feel so bad before. So it really freaked me out that abstinence came with feeling so lousy.

For an addict without a pot-bellied stove, feeling so lousy was like being in the mother of all blizzards without a parka. I knew freezing to death (in my case death meant going back to using), was just around the corner and it was coming really fast.

Then, just when I thought my condition could not get any worse, it did.

Very suddenly, the overall feeling lousy started to separate into pieces. In no particular order of how bad I felt, describing each, hopefully will be helpful if you are going through or about to go through the same experience of being abstinent for a while. Reading this might also be helpful to those who care about you and don't understand what is happening to you.

I will start with anxiety. It is a familiar word, but what is meant by it is not well understood. I certainly did not understand the meaning even when it became my daily companion. It came and went as it pleased, at first, always unexpectedly for no particular reason I could see. Then a pattern started to show itself.

I became overwhelmed with anxiety whenever I wanted or was expected to do something that was even just a little out of my comfort zone. The problem, I slowly came to realize, was that mostly nothing was ever expected of me in the past. To be clear, nothing constructive, acceptable or desirable was ever expected of me. All that was ever expected of me was to be a screw-up. And I was always very good at that. Therefore, I had almost no confidence in my ability to do or accomplish anything worthwhile. Very good reasons, I believe, to be anxious. For example, I dreaded speaking, especially at AA meetings. I dreaded meeting new people and I dreaded doing anything new or different. Always, I feared screwing up and feared that screwing up would literally destroy me. Caring about what I do and how I do it for the first time in my life came at a huge price.

The very close cousin to my anxiety, always lurking in the

shadows and jumping out to scare the living crap out of me were 'panic attacks'. Because the attacks were so severe and always occurred, so it seemed, when I had to do something important, they really messed up my ability to get things done, especially to be a reliable parent.

The panic attacks can be best described as anxiety on several tons of steroids. Times when I was driving are probably the best examples. You are probably surprised I have a car and can drive. These are the benefits of being abstinent. But back to describing a panic attack while driving.

It was a rather ordinary, clear day. I was approaching a bridge on a familiar road when all of a sudden, my heart started to pound, my legs turned into wobbly jelly, and I became drenched in sweat. In my mind, like a repeating recorded warning, I kept thinking I was going to lose control, drive off the bridge and die. Somehow, I managed to pull myself together enough to cross the bridge and pull off the road. In a parking lot, at full stop, I sobbed and shook uncontrollably. It took some time to regain my composure and only then was I able to drive where I was going.

The thing about the panic attack was that, logically, there was nothing to be afraid of but I still felt very emotional as if I were actually going to die. My brain truly believing this was putting my body into action mode, like the heart pounding, the blood rushing to where it's needed like my legs, and my body sweating because of all this action going on.

The panic attacks and just generally feeling anxious could happen at any time, mostly with very little warning. Even though on some level, I knew these to be irrational reactions, it did not matter; they came upon me anyway. As you can imagine, I was pretty much out of commission. I could not be counted on to keep my word to do sometimes the simplest thing. Of course, this just added to my feeling bad.

The next, close relative of anxiety and panic attack is fear. Not just any fear but a real, intense fear. When I felt it, it was like someone was going to kill me or I was just going to die. At times, even during some minor unpleasant interaction, the fear was so intense that I went into an automatic, out-of-control overreaction, self-preservational, aggressive mode. I would become like one of those very irritating small dogs that viciously bark at anything and everything because it is afraid. Needless to say, I was not pleasant to be around. People said behind my back and to my face: "What's up with her (you)?" pretty much all the time.

You are probably anticipating, and correctly at that, that all of these horribly negative emotions made me terribly sad. There was no joy or quality to my life. My only escape at the time came through the few times I could sleep for a few hours. I was getting very close to giving up on my abstinence. In fact, I started to think about getting back together with my old reliable friends, alcohol and whatever drug I could get my hands on.

By this time in my abstinence, I sort of had an AA sponsor, a guy who I believed had his shit together. I trusted him to help me through the tough parts. So, as is the AA way of doing things, I shared how I was feeling, and especially that I was getting close to freezing to death in this blizzard-like life of new sobriety. Freezing to death for us folk without pot-bellied stoves is going back to using, and we do freeze to death without the external heat that comes from the AA fellowship. While I was not about to freeze to death, since I was going to a meeting almost every night, it sure felt like I was. I wanted, and I believed I needed, serious help.

My sponsor made two welcomed and comforting comments. One, that my condition was not uncommon among the recently sober or abstinent. Two, that he knew someone who could help me get through this rough patch that comes with recent sobriety.

For a curious person, I was not at all curious about anything he said or what he meant by getting help from someone. All I was interested in, was that there was help for me, and that he could hook me up with this help right away. Does this sound familiar to those of you without pot-bellied stoves?

CHAPTER 2
If It Sounds Too Good
To Be True, It Is

All people, especially those like me, without a pot-bellied stove, want, often demand, quick and easy fixes to our problems. Anyone offering such a thing is always most welcome, no questions asked.

So, when the 'promise' of help was offered, I asked no questions. I was exhausted physically and mentally by the work I was doing to get and stay sober. I did not have the energy to take responsibility for one more thing – those lousy emotions that come to the surface when not using for a while. I needed and wanted an out for my previously avoided/buried emotional problems. While in the past, the problems were never fixed, they were just avoided. This time, so I believed, a professional was actually going to cure the things that were bothering me.

Imagine my delight when I found out that the person who was going to help me was a physician-specialist in psychiatry. Since the specialist was a medical doctor, not one of those Ph.D.'s, I figured my emotional problems were being caused by some physical illness, not by me being a screw-up.

I was feeling panicky, anxious, afraid, and sad because I was physically ill. After all, so I reasoned, medical doctors treat the physically ill, not screw-ups. Just like when I had to take a pill to cure an infection, I expected the doctor to give me a pill to cure what was making me feel bad.

Just when I thought my delight could not get any better, when I met the psychiatrist, I learned that she had the ability and authority to label me, (diagnose), and based on that label, had a specific pill to give me to make me feel better. I will come back to this, "make me feel better", several times because the words are critically important to the point of this chapter.

But back to what happened. You can hardly blame me for wanting to believe that my mental and emotional, negative states were being caused by physical problems. My stomach was always queasy. I had bouts of diarrhea, followed by periods of constipation. At times, I had difficulty breathing, could not catch my breath and then, sometimes, I shook like a leaf or my heart raced as if I was running for my life.

It never occurred to me at that time to ask which came first, the mental and emotional or the physical problems. I was simply too focused on getting a quick and easy fix without losing my hard-earned, sustained sobriety.

Given my focus, it is not surprising how I interpreted what I heard. The pill was going to make me feel better; no mess, no fuss, nothing for me to do but to take it. Nothing else mattered. It never occurred to me to ask questions and certainly the psychiatrist said nothing about what was causing me to feel so bad emotionally or even physically. My main concern was that the pill was going to make me feel better. Why would I have been interested in anything else?

For example, I had not noticed that the label (diagnosis) the psychiatrist applied to me was not based on bloodwork or scan results. The label chosen was based on what I had said but, as I learned later, meant that I had a biochemical imbalance. Why this was not confirmed by some physical test never occurred to me at the time.

I was blinded by the easy quick-fix light.

Here, it is important for me not to be misleading. I don't want to give the impression that the psychiatrist suggested or somehow implied the pill was going to cure me. There was no mention of a cure, only that the pill "will make you feel better". Because I was only interested in getting relief from my horrible mental and emotional state, I asked no questions.

Relief, however, never came. Instead, my dance with the psychiatrist became a huge experiment at a cost I did not anticipate or sign up for. Like street drugs, cigarettes, and alcohol, a prescribed psychiatric drug takes some getting used to. Like all drugs, the initial first pill was a strange chemical to my body, which it naturally treated as something to get rid of. So this full-scale war was created in my body as it worked to kick the drug out and the drug worked to stay in. The drug, being a synthetic intoxicant, was more powerful and won the battle but not without casualties or side effects.

Because of a side effect, the drug, one pill, became drugs, more than one pill; a pill for this and a pill for that, sometimes a higher dose for one and a lower dose for another. One pill replaced another, and sometimes more pills were added to the list. I was not doing well, and the promise of "this will help" was not being delivered. My hope was slowly but surely being destroyed.

Since this was a completely new dance to me, and I was regularly attending AA meetings, I eagerly and openly talked to others. It did not take long to discover others were having almost the same experiences. This information justified my belief that I was getting the right kind of help, and I just had to put up with the war in my body for a while.

Once the side effects (like dry mouth or swollen tongue), of the pills decreased, their effect on my brain started to kick in. It was strange, freaky and, most of all, very unusual.

I felt increasingly more sedated to the point that I cared less and less about anything and everything. Before, while smoking pot, I was just mellow without a care in the world. The added punch to the psychiatric drugs was something else. The added 'value' was that I started not to care if I lived or died.

Before some of my friends got to this way of feeling, a few had very serious physical problems; problems far worse than the emotional problems that caused them to ask for help from a psychiatrist in the first place. One of my friends even died from the side effects of the drugs she was prescribed.

That was not going to be me.

A very delightfully promising source of help turned out to be a disastrous experience for me and my friends. Driven by good, healthy survival instincts, I went into my research mode and easily found a lot of scary information about psychiatry and its so-called medicine.

There, for the curious looking, I found out that the pills I was prescribed were forms of synthetic sedatives. They were not curing or fixing anything, they were just sedating me to the point that I dangerously did not care about anything. This was not what I expected from the "this will help" approach. Clearly, I was so wrong.

CHAPTER 3
Involuntary Intoxication

've heard people say that, "ignorance is bliss". Well, it's not, especially when it comes to your mental and physical well-being. In fact, you could pay a very high price for your blissful ignorance; the price could very well be your life. I escaped the grim reaper, but not before some seriously bad shit happened to me. I was saved by my considerable instinct to survive. Even when I was stoned, I always sensed danger so I knew what it felt like to be in danger when stoned, and I was stoned on the prescribed pills and in danger.

I can't explain all this without some seriously big words in this chapter. So, get ready. I will, however, define the words as best I can.

Without even having to read anything, the first lesson I learned in this brief, nasty dance with psychiatry was how important it is to really know and understand to what you are agreeing. For example, before a surgery, everyone signs a consent form after what is going to be done is explained. This was not done with me or my friends when we were prescribed a psychiatric drug. There was no informed consent form for any of us to sign. In a very matter of fact way, I was simply expected to take a pill for my diagnosis (label) because it would make me "feel better". I should have asked for a definition of "feel better", and at what cost but I did not.

In the past, when I bought alcohol or drugs, I expected, in fact, wanted to get high. The technical word for it is 'intoxicated'. However, I did not realize that when I filled the psychiatrist's prescription, I was doing the same thing: buying a pill to get intoxicated.

Later, I learned that there is an actual phrase for what was being done to me. It is called "involuntary intoxication". This means that my brain was being chemically altered not to be in its normal state of sobriety. Sobriety which I achieved and was working so hard to maintain, was being messed with, and I had no idea that it was happening. My psychiatrist was getting me stoned (sedated) without my permission or knowledge. Think about that for a while.

So, stoned I got with all that comes with it. For example, I had strange and weird thoughts as well as the behaviours that went with it. I became obsessed with ending the strange, buzzing sensation in my head. Then I got desperate to end it, thinking that the only way to do it would be to kill myself. Stoned in this way, I also experienced a new and unfamiliar feeling: I did not care if I lived or died. And if I was going to kill myself, I believed, it would not be right to leave my baby boy behind. So, I was thinking I should, at the same time, kill him thus taking him with me.

At my core, I have an intense drive to survive, and this instinct forced me out of the haze into reality, which started my gradual putting an end to this nasty dance with psychiatry.

Before I go any further, I should tell you that when I first took the prescribed pills, they actually made me "feel better". I thought the doctor was right. The pill was doing what she said it would. Of course, it was and, as I learned later, the antidepressant, like all such drugs, is really just a sedative. And, at least in the beginning, being sedated, getting mellow, can be quite pleasant. But like a frog who does not know it is being slowly boiled to death, I was completely unaware what else the prescribed drug was doing to me. I was slipping into an unreal world, an altered state of mind and completely unaware of it happening. Since I was not expecting to be stoned on, intoxicated without my informed consent, I believed my altered state of mind to be a good thing, especially initially. Later, I learned this, too, has a name: "medication spellbinding".

When my instinct to survive kicked in and I had had enough of being made weird by sedatives, there were more lessons to be learned. Like from alcohol and street drugs, you can go through horrible withdrawal between taking pills and certainly when you decide to stop them. Going through withdrawal for illegal and legal psychiatrist-prescribed drugs is not pretty, and is the time a person is most likely to do something dangerously out of character. Incidentally, the same applies when you are building up the concentration of a legal or illegal drug in your body. Curious how you never read about this in any report on investigation into a horrendous, murderous, out-of-character rampage by a person with so-called 'mental health problems' who is 'under psychiatric care'.

Another effect of the pill(s) that scared me was a growing agitation, like a wild mushroom; a restlessness I had never experienced before. Yes, I was always hyper as a kid, but never like this. Literally, I could not sit still. I could not stop myself from pacing like a stressed, caged animal in a bad old-fashioned zoo. More manic than not, I had so much energy that I believed I could carry out the killing of my son, then myself. This really freaked me out. It was another bell ringing to get my attention. For those of you who like fancy concepts, words that have a specific meaning, this drug-created state of agitation is called, 'akathisia' in the books. In that big book on the psychiatrist's desk, there is even a warning about when you get like this: "Akathisia may be associated with dysphoria (a painful emotion), irritability (overreacting with anger or hostility), aggression or suicide attempts". Then, the book goes on to warn that akathisia can lead to "worsening of psychotic symptoms or behavioural dyscontrol (being out of control). Just remember, the state of akathisia was caused by the prescribed drug in the first place.

There are more side effects created by these drugs. The worst, because it cannot be reversed, is something called 'tardive dyskinesia'. This fancy term refers to disfiguring grimaces and tics (facial twitches) - you guessed it - caused by a psychiatrist-prescribed pill. If a person is really unlucky, which thankfully I was not, the side effect also could include abnormal arm, leg and neck movements. If a person is really, really unlucky, the pill(s) could affect the muscles involved in speaking, swallowing and breathing.

What was starting to happen to me and to my AA friends with similar issues you can see for yourself in neighbourhoods where there are many lodging homes whose residents walk about aimlessly. Their strange posture, how they shuffle or walk, and their facial distortions are the side effects that I have been describing. Many, if not all, are beyond the point of no return. And they got there without signing up for it or knowing where they were headed. Because initially, they were "medication spellbound" they did not hear the warning bells as I was lucky enough to hear. Perhaps, when they heard them they did not know what the bells meant. Regardless, those poor souls are lost forever, and thankfully, likely don't even know it.

You may be wondering why I have been writing pill

with the (s). The reason is that I and others like me are prescribed only one pill for a very brief period of time. Most of the time, I was prescribed several, and the dose of each changed frequently.

Last but by no means least, I want to end this chapter by sharing what I learned about the physical effects the prescribed drugs have on a person's body. We all know that constant drinking of alcohol destroys the liver; it is called cirrhosis. Essentially, the liver wears out from constantly processing the poison otherwise known as ethanol, which is the key ingredient in all booze. If that happens with alcoholic drinks, what happens when the body is under the influence of (is intoxicated by) psychiatrist-prescribed pills? A good question to be sure.

I already talked about the irreversible distortions of the body and face. There are even more irreversible effects as, for example, in the brain. I read that the brain scan of people who shut out the real world and create in their head a world of their own is different from people who don't do that. But I also read the difference is cause by the psychiatrist-prescribed pill(s), rather than it being the cause of people's very screwed-up ways of reacting to very difficult, crazy-making conditions in their life. Taking a prescribed drug that causes permanent 'brain damage', in my way of thinking, is a very high price to pay just for wanting "to feel better". You would think it would be better to change what is causing the person to mentally escape their shit life, like mine used to be.

Everyone knows about dry mouth being a side effect of many drugs, including those prescribed by psychiatrists. It should be of no surprise therefore, that constipation is a common side effect of many prescribed pills. My friend Mary suffered from it almost as soon as she started taking the first psychiatrist- prescribed pill. As another friend likes to say, "if you don't shit, you die". That is exactly what happened to Mary. In a following chapter, I will describe in great detail her ordeal. No one should ever go through what was done to her. And it was done to her, even though she did not sign up for it.

To summarise, I did not sign up to be involuntarily, without my 'informed consent', made intoxicated. I just wanted to 'feel better', that's all. It was a good thing I had enough remaining sense to stop the nasty dancing before it was too late. I had enough sense to ask what exactly the pill was supposed to do. To my surprise, I discovered, mostly by reading, that the pills simply sedate you. Being sedated at first, can be pleasant for you and those around you. But there is a huge price to pay for the short-lived relief from life's unavoidable problems.

CHAPTER 4
Ask Questions

My experience with psychiatry was similar to that of many of my friends in AA. At first, we all believed ourselves to be in good scientific hands. We were all impressed by the big book (DSM5) that gave a label to how we were feeling and behaving. We were equally impressed that the label came with the name of a 'medication' specifically made to make people with a specific, labelled problem "feel better".

Very quickly, however, the wheels started to fall off our wagon of hope. The first wheel that fell off was the same for all of us, and we were equally responsible for it happening. No one, including myself, had the good sense to ask, "What do you mean, it will make me feel better?" We also did not know to ask, "at what cost (i.e. side effects) will the pill make me feel better?". Not asking the second question was more excusable because most people do not ask about the side effects of a pill they are prescribed. And whatever paper is given with the prescription warning of side effects, who reads the small print, understands or remembers that stuff? Very few, I think. But, at the very least, we should have asked for a definition of "feel better" and how that was going to be accomplished.

As usual, I got to thinking, which always ends up with me reading. My experience and that of my AA friends all started to make some sense. I say some sense, because the area of 'mental health' and psychiatry's role in it is a very complex subject that has at least two sides to it. One side, mostly the establishment, is all in favour of psychiatry and its partner, the psycho-pharmaceutical (drug makers) industry. The other side, much less well known, is highly critical of the specialty and the drugs it prescribes. While a small and scholarly group, it is very vocal about its position.

What I want to do in this chapter, therefore, is to give enough information to stir up your curiosity and interest to read and educate yourself before you get to dancing with a psychiatrist.

To begin, since people started to write about stuff, there has been a debate about how to understand behaviour that is troublesome. There seems to be two broad sides to the debate: one side calls it an illness; the other side simply calls it bad behaviour. At one time, medical directors of what were called asylums believed 'insanity' to be a disease of the brain caused by social conditions in a person's environment. As you can imagine, the idea turned out not to be very popular. No one was eager to accept responsibility for creating environments that make people 'crazy'.

Psychiatry started to emerge as a specialty gaining in popularity, essentially because a biological cause of 'insanity' was discovered. Syphilis in its last stages was found to cause muscle and nerve damage, which makes people behave very strangely. If there is one biological cause of madness (strange behaviour) it was reasoned, there must be others, and it is just a matter of time before others are found. But less than ten others have been found, described and given a label in that big book (DSM5) relied on by psychiatrists.

Even the association to which psychiatrists belong (APA), has admitted that the search for a biological cause of insanity has not panned out. Sadly for all of us, most family physicians and physician-specialists in psychiatry did not get this memo. They continue to speak of chemical imbalance without any physical evidence of it, and they continue to use chemical substances to make things right.

This then brings me to tell you what I learned about the trick bag full of pills that psychiatrists prescribe to balance those chemical imbalances. The pills can be put into two groups. Most are sedatives and some are uppers (stimulants).

As an addict who was addicted, I know all too well that intoxicating chemicals affect different people differently. Also, I know all too well that the same, intoxicating chemical can have from time to time different effects on the same person depending on the amount taken. The challenge, therefore, of using illegal and prescribed, legal drugs is the same: It is to find the right drug in the right amount, to create the desired effect. We experimented on the street just as physicians experiment with what and how much they prescribe "to make you feel better". While this kind of experimentation can be dangerous both on the street and in the psychiatrist's office, unfortunately it does go on at both places. As far as I can figure, there are two reasons for this. The first is us and our desperate need to escape feeling lousy. The second is the money to be made by supplying us with illegal and legal drugs, including the drug otherwise known as alcohol. The drug manufacturers must have decided to get into the action that has made and continues to make drug dealers and alcohol distillers very rich.

As the saying goes, if you want to understand motivation, just follow the money.

During my curious search for information and then

writing about what I found, I also learned something about myself. It would seem that I am also an idealistic person. I'm idealistic because I am expecting/hoping that my nasty experiences and those of my friends will cause you to take a step back before you jump from the frying pan of street drugs into the fire of psychiatrist-prescribed legal drugs. We have all seen overdose deaths, especially recently from opioids and harm to the liver, stomach, intestines, skin, and other parts of the body caused by street drugs. Similar damage is caused by prescribed drugs. What makes this kind of harm worse, is that no one is expecting it or signs up for it, willingly.

So, if "this will make you feel better" is offered to you, do not hesitate to ask for a definition. Also, do not hesitate to ask for a print-out of the drug's side effects. When you get it, read it. By reading it and perhaps doing some research of your own, you just might find out that the drug can be toxic to the heart, interfere with how you process the food you need to stay alive, cause you to gain weight or get diabetes, high blood pressure or increase your cholesterol.

I am concluding this hopefully scary chapter by urging you to ask how long you need to take the prescribed drug, and what will it do to your body and brain if you take it for six months, a year or even longer.

The mother of all questions to ask a psychiatrist when you are offered a pill, is what alternative 'treatments' are available to improve how you think, feel, and behave. If no alternative is identified or offered, don't walk out of the office. Run!

CHAPTER 5
Worst Case Scenarios

Since my nasty dance with psychiatry and all my research, I have been especially aware that violent individuals shooting or bombing many others are often described as having a 'mental health problem'. I have also become equally aware that seldom, if ever, the investigations of a violent, out of control individual do not include looking into the person's mental health issues. For example, no information is provided and analysed about who was 'treating' the person, what was the nature of the treatment and what, if any, medication was the person starting, taking for a while, or coming off.

These are important questions as I learned from my own experiences and from watching others. For sure, starting or getting off a psychiatrist prescribed drug can make you feel not like yourself, or worse. If you research this, even a little, you will quickly find out some very scary stuff.

The first thing you will find is that, for good reasons, the American Food and Drug Administration (FDA) makes drug companies put some very scary warnings on their products. For example, every antidepressant label has a "Warning: Clinical Worsening and Suicide Risk" section. The warning applies to both children and adults. It continues, "anxiety, agitation, panic attacks, insomnia, irritability, hostility, aggressiveness, impulsivity, akathisia (psychomotor restlessness), hypomania and mania" could be caused or made worse by taking the drug. What all this means, I believe, is that the conditions listed in the warning could be made worse or be caused by the drug, not the person's environment, emotions, ways of reasoning or are the later-life, negative consequences of early life-horrible experiences. I was most shocked to read the part that antidepressants can cause people to be violent or suicidal.

Pretty risky business taking a psychiatrist prescribed drug, but millions of people take them all the time. Like me, people don't ask questions and certainly seldom, if ever, read the warnings that come with every prescription.

Why anyone, including myself, would take such risks is very easy to answer. In the beginning of my nasty dance, I did not know better and my friends were also unaware. If we had been properly warned, which we were not, none of us would have heard it because we were so focused on an easy, quick fix to feeling lousy.

The reality that many others have similarly fallen victim to the promise of an easy, quick fix does not make me feel any better about how I agreed to dance with the psychiatrist.

Peter Breggin is a psychiatrist I found by looking. He writes about the dangers of getting involved with people in his profession whose only tool for 'helping' are pills. In his books, he provides many examples of people doing strange and awful things when getting on, being on, or getting off a psycho-pharmaceutical drug. And everyone should know that not only psychiatrists prescribe them. Well-intentioned, but not well informed family physicians can, and do, also prescribe them.

In his books, Breggin describes real cases of drug-caused, bizarre thinking that lead to equally bizarre behaviour. In one case, a man on a psychiatrist- prescribed drug to 'treat' his depression almost kills a policeman in the act of trying to get his gun with which to kill himself. In another case, a family physician- prescribed drug, also for depression, drove a young girl to compulsive states of violence, during which she almost killed her mother. In the saddest case, what he recounts all happened in thirty days; a boy not yet twelve years old, was diagnosed, was prescribed an antidepressant, and shortly after committed suicide.

Breggin describes many other horrible cases but these few examples should be enough to both scare you and make you curious to find out more. You should also know that there are many more highly-trained professionals like Breggin who are just as critical of biological psychiatry and their primary tool, psycho-pharmaceutical drugs.

While many people successfully sue psychiatrists for malpractice, most interesting to me was to find out that there are successful lawsuits against the medical schools for how they trained psychiatrists. Of course, the outcome of these lawsuits are not well publicized and often settlements are reached before a public trial. It's best to keep these things quiet, I am guessing.

Not all critics of psychiatry and their reliance on drugs blame individuals for the harm that they cause. Some, who write about such things, blame the "system". The idea of a 'system' to my mind is very complex, but I think it sort of means a runaway train that needs lots and lots of money to keep going.

The lucky among us see the light before it's too late, and get out. As I already warned, getting out can be very tricky and sometimes downright dangerous. This was the case with

Mary. I still shudder when I think it could have been me. To honour her life, therefore, and to inform the vulnerable to think long and hard before then agree to dance with psychiatry, I will end this chapter by telling her story.

Mary was a very capable divorced mother of two children. She shared parenting responsibly with the father and held down a demanding full-time job. Like me, she also was the product of very negative early-life conditions. The difference between us, was that Mary appeared to be coping with it all. She was coping even with her divorce.

We knew Mary she was drinking, but none of us knew how much. To her absolute credit, Mary knew she was drinking "too much" and decided to stop. Also, to her absolute credit, Mary was honest enough with herself to know she could not get and stay sober by herself. She instinctively knew she needed the AA program and started to attend regularly.

By the time she reached her first anniversary of sobriety, the underlying issues from which she hid by drinking were all at the surface. She had never felt as bad before. Unpredictable, intense panic attacks were especially problematic for her. As was the expectation in the AA program she talked about it openly and often. Her sort of AA sponsor listened, validated her emotional and mental pain and, most importantly, counselled her about a way out. The way out for Mary, according to the sponsor, was to see a psychiatrist, who he said would be able to help her. She jumped at the chance of getting help that did not require much from her. She already had a lot on her plate. She did not want another project. It would have been too much on top of everything else she was already doing. So, psychiatry it was, and she eagerly took the quick, easy "fix pill" that was prescribed for her. Similar to the rest of us, the one pill quickly became more and there was much experimentation with the amounts she was prescribed.

As I described before, psychiatric drugs can have all sorts of effects on your mind and body. Mary's bad luck was that the drugs she was prescribed dried her up. They gave her dry mouth and seriously constipated her. No truer words have been spoken: "if you don't shit, you die". Whatever efforts were made to help her, nothing worked. Mary's guts became full of hard-as-cement crap. Because the crap was hard and sharp, it punctured several holes in her intestine, releasing toxic shit into her body. She was hospitalized and put into a medically-created coma for many days just to keep her alive; kept her alive they did, but not for long.

Mary was never the same after she was discharged from the hospital. Her looks went seriously downhill. She went grey and started to walk with a cane. A beautiful woman, almost overnight, became a children's fairy tale, forest-dwelling, old character. She never went back to the psychiatrist, she never went back to work and she stopped going to her AA meetings. The period from the beginning to the end of her short, nasty dance with psychiatry was just over a year. The tragedy is, that only a few of us have learned anything from her experience and death. Probably the psychiatrist is carrying on just the same as before.

No one person is responsible for Mary's completely avoidable death. We are all responsible. We are responsible for our collective ignorance, for not asking the important questions and for handing over responsibility for our well-being in exchange for a promise of a quick and easy fix expressed as, "this will make you feel better".

CHAPTER 6
"Mental Health" Professionals

Addicts, like me, especially need to know who the various players are in the mental health professions, what they believe, and based on their beliefs, what they actually do. Since virtually everyone, at one time or another, from what I see, could use help with their personal issues, we could all be better informed than we are about whom to call. I, and many of my friends, learned the hard way about what the various disciplines do, and why. Mary died learning the lesson. Writing this chapter, I'm hoping, will save others from having to go through our experiences.

To begin, I do not like the word 'health' when talking about my state of mind or how I am feeling emotionally. The word gives the impression that there is something going on physically, that what I am thinking and feeling is caused by something physical, biological or organic. In other words, something that is not naturally in my body. This way of thinking then leads to the conclusion that a physician, a medical doctor, is the only person who can help. Not true. There is nothing physical going on to cause most bad behaviour, so

I learned in my curious search for understanding. No one, including me, catches 'something' from a door- knob to make them behave badly.

What about genetics? You might ask. My parents and my grandparents were all screw-ups so that must prove that they, and I, inherited our messed-up ways. So far, however, no one has discovered a gene that causes bad behaviour, and those who study people behaving badly all say we learn to act from watching how people closest to us cope with life. While I did not ask to be born into a messed-up family, while I did not ask to be messed up by the lousy environment in which they raised me, and while I did not ask to be deprived of 'empathic nurturance' with which to make a warm, pot-bellied stove, I am nevertheless the not so proud outcome of all of the above. Since I have the consequences, I own them. I am, as I see it, responsible for them, which means I am responsible for finding out what kind of help I need and who is best able to give it. For me, this part of the journey started with better words than 'mental health' to describe my issues. I'll take dysfunctional, maladaptive, badly behaved, messed-up thinker or any label other than that of suffering from 'mental health' issues.

Sadly, the currently popular and most acceptable way of describing people like me is that we have 'mental health' issues. That is one of the reasons why physician-specialists in psychiatry are kings of the castle, on top of the pile, make the most money, and are given the greatest status and the greatest respect around the world. How this came about seems to me to have been caused by the so-called perfect storm.

The perfect storm includes people that do not want to accept responsibility for screwing up their kids, and psychiatrists that hunt for a biological cause of madness in order to be respected in their own medical profession.

As physicians searching for a biological cause of madness, it makes perfect sense for them to partner up with drug manufacturers who could then 'cure' the biological cause of bad behaviour. Inspite of finding only a handful of physical causes for very specific types of madness, the partnership between the two continues. It is very much alive and well, simply because it handsomely pays off for both of them. As for the public, the pay-off is not so good. In fact for far too many, it is harmful. It is harmful for reasons already discussed and for reasons I will describe in the next chapter.

To be precise, biological psychiatry believes that bad, dysfunctional, maladaptive, in short, messed up behaviour is caused by physical abnormalities and that these can be fixed with one psycho-pharmaceutical drug or more. So, if you want to be legally sedated to the state that you don't care about anything, including hearing voices, this is the discipline for you. As a sober addict, working to stay that way, the last thing I needed to deal with my negative emotions and thoughts was getting intoxicated with a psychiatrist-prescribed drug and suffering the side effects. If I ever get so desperate for relief, I'll just go back to drinking and using street drugs. At least I know the harm they cause.

Next on the list of establishment-assigned status, is the discipline of psychology, specifically clinical psychologists. In the last ten or more years, I read that some or perhaps most clinical psychologists want to be like psychiatrists. While their doctor title is a Ph. D., they want to be able to diagnose using the same book (DSM5) that psychiatrists use. Some also want to prescribe the same drugs after taking two years of special training. Psychiatry, of course, is opposed to this. They do not want the competition, but got it anyway. In most places, psychology is given the authority to use the same diagnostic book and labels as psychiatry. To my shock and horror, I also discovered that in New Mexico and Louisiana, clinical psychologists can prescribe the same pills as psychiatrists. By now, there could be more places where psychology is doing this.

It was difficult therefore, to figure out what beliefs shape what psychologists do. Most, I think, focus on helping people change how they think, and as a result behave, which then affects their emotions. Their training is to focus on the person, and to use 'psychological tests' to help figure out the nature and intensity of a person's problem(s). They believe that a person's problems are caused by how they think, behave and feel. What they do, therefore, is focus on helping a person change or modify one or all of the above.

Clinical social workers believe in a bigger picture of how people function. They believe that a person's environment, which includes people and conditions, greatly influences how they cope with life's challenges. They are trained to examine the person in the context of their life, how they live, where they live, who they live with, the nature of their relationships, and what life experiences have shaped who they have become.

What clinical social workers do, therefore, is focus on modifying or making better conditions in the person's environment. Mostly, they partner up with a person to figure out how to change things in the environment, in order to help the person think, behave, and emotionally feel better.

In addition to these three disciplines (I am careful not to call them 'mental health' professionals), there are registered psychotherapists, couple therapists, and therapists who 'treat' the whole family. As with all important commitments, you need to shop around to find the person with whom you are comfortable, and in whom you have confidence to be able to help you in the way you need help.

As you can see, what Mary did not know, her naïve trust, first in her AA sponsor, then in her physician-specialist in psychiatry, she paid for with her life. My ignorance and the ignorance of many friends also harmed us but luckily we got out just in time.

What remains to be said is that after all this nasty dancing with psychiatry, I have a whole new respect for how powerful the influence of the establishment is on all of our lives. This influence equally affects the psychiatrist who 'treated' Mary, and the AA sponsor who took her there. Neither intended to harm her. Both were only doing what they knew, and what they believed in. Sadly, both did not know what they did not know. While we cannot possibly know everything about everything, you can bet that from then on I will investigate and research everything before I agree to anything. I still make impulsive decisions, mostly about buying shoes but not about what I put into my body. I try to take my time, do some research, and make decisions that are well informed.

As a result of blindly trusting the establishment and almost ending up like Mary – dead – I got to thinking. I started to wonder why so many people want to belong to the establishment and why so many people, like me, Mary and others, so readily trust what it has to offer.

Thinking about this is the reason I decided to write a four-book trilogy. Yes, I know a trilogy is three, but I am in good company, since the classic, The *Hitchhikers Guide to the Galaxy*, is also a trilogy of four books. For now, I just want to touch on the highlights of the fourth book, the major theme of which is the squandering of the gift of potential by settling and getting stuck at the reference/tribal stage of cognitive development.

For example, if you think about it, the establishment very rich, or the 1% is nothing more than just another tribe;

albeit very powerful tribe, one with specific beliefs, values, and ways of doing things. Most people are born into it, and the rest "perspire" (that's a deliberate mistake) to get into it. Those who perspire to get into it, protect it, justify it, make excuses for what it does because they expect to be in it "any day now". So, they buy lottery tickets or work their buns off, hoping to have enough money to be able to buy the right cars, live in the right neighbourhood in a big enough house, and belong to the right clubs to be accepted into this small, elite tribe. However, unlike most other tribes, who recruit new members, the establishment or 1% tribe wants to remain exclusive, and they achieve it by keeping people out.

Mary's sponsor sober for some time and, as a result, doing well financially, I believer was *perspiring* to become a member of the establishment tribe. So, he did what most people do in that tribe, trust the most highly regarded and expensive, so-called mental health professional, the psychiatrist. As a perspirant (a word I made up) wannabe, he would never have thought of taking Mary to a psychologist, let alone a social worker. It had to be a medical specialist in psychiatry, since he observed the successful establishment types all doing similar things. I say again, therefore, blaming is not a very useful thing to do. The sponsor really believed he was doing the right thing. Of course, the psychiatrist also believed in the value of involuntarily intoxicating Mary.

Instead of blaming, we would all be better off if we learned not to trust as easily, and to be a lot more inclined to get better informed by doing research. At the very least, after doing research, no one could ask in amazement when the shit hits the fan: "What were you thinking?"

CHAPTER 7
All Drugs Are Business

In this chapter, I am going to write briefly about the history of drug use, and a great deal about drugs that people who behave strangely are prescribed by physician-specialists in psychiatry, family physicians and, in at least two American states, specially trained psychologists. I learned a great deal in a short time just by reading. You should do the same, especially before, not after, you are made intoxicated without your permission.

Getting intoxicated, however, is no new experience for human beings. We have been doing it since time immemorial. Humans have been forever smoking hallucinogens in the jungles of South America, Africa, and Asia in search of a 'spiritual' experience. In some places, people lick frogs for a similar effect or eat 'magic mushrooms' with the same purpose in mind. Most people have heard of opium dens in parts of the Orient exported to other countries and written about in old cheesy mystery novels. Many, however, have forgotten that *Coca Cola* was originally laced with cocaine to give the drinker that boost, and that *7Up* originally had lithium as an ingredient to treat gout, which at one time was more common than now. The bottom line is that human beings have never been opposed to consuming what we know clearly now to have been 'snake-oil' remedies. My humble conclusion, based on my brief but intense research, is that not much has changed when it comes to chemically treating mental and emotional problems. The only real difference is the packaging of the snake oil and what we call it.

The following is a summary of what is written about psychiatric drugs. Most of it comes from books written by Peter Breggin and his colleagues. On purpose, I am not calling psychiatric drugs medication. Usually, a medicine cures something and, therefore, is good for you, although according to Mary Poppins, a little sugar sometimes helps to make it go down.

There are at least five categories, families or groups of drugs. They are: antidepressants, tranquilizers (including sleeping pills), antipsychotic drugs (neuroleptics), mood stabilizers, and stimulants. Curiously, it was not easy to find clear information on these drugs even in what professionals critical of psychiatry write. Being stubborn as a mule came in real handy researching this topic.

There are at least 18 different types of antidepressants, and they are made of many different types of chemicals. There is much written about what chemical effect they produce in the body. For example, the drugs block dopamine and/or histamine or alpha – 1 adrenergic receptors, noradrenaline and serotonin reuptake are also blocked. What these chemicals are in the body, how what they do is measured in a depressed person, as well as what they have to do with a person feeling depressed is a whole other matter. At the end of my reading about antidepressants, what I learned is that most are sedatives, and some have a mild stimulating effect.

Most importantly, I discovered by reading that there is nothing physical in the body that is a sign or cause of depression. That's why there is no bloodwork or scan images that can 'diagnose' it. So, all that stuff about chemical blockers and uptakes seems to be about what happens once you are depressed. Regardless of all this action, according to studies, whether a person takes antidepressants or sugar pills, there is no difference in how they feel. And if sedated enough, people stop caring about what was making them depressed. This is a very familiar state, and one I was constantly chasing after when using.

These psychiatrist-prescribed antidepressants, however, can have toxic effects on the body and the mind, in some people even increase or cause suicidal and violent tendencies.

Taking pills to 'cure' depression, or to 'make better' how you feel, as you can see, is not such a good idea. In fact, for most of us, it is a very bad deal. If you are tempted to try, at the very least do your research, and do it with eyes wide open.

The second group of drugs I want to briefly describe are the tranquilizers, in particular, sleeping pills. They are sort of more powerful sedatives, but sound just as harmless until you discover that they belong to the family of drugs known as benzodiazepines. Now, this name sounds a lot more sinister for good reasons. Sleeping pills are all tranquilizers, the same as pills prescribed for anxiety or panic attacks. Most troubling, especially for an addict like me, is that the tranquilizers have similar effects to alcohol (probably also marijuana), and we all know what stupid, dysfunctional things people can do when intoxicated or under the influence. Also, I remember passing out when drunk or stoned on pot and then suddenly waking up when the drug-caused effect wore off. Passing out from street or legal drugs is not the same as a restful, rejuvenating night of sleep. It is certainly not a good long-term strategy for coping with what is troubling you. Although, I was glad to have a tranquilizer prescribed briefly for my mom after my father died and a sleeping pill in hospital for me when the noise kept me awake.

I am hoping that by now you are recognizing a theme. Apart from stimulants, the other prescribed drugs all look to be nothing more than different types of sedatives or tranquilizers. Prozac, Xanax, Klonopin, Valium and Ativan, to name just a few, are substances that sedate/tranqualize you. As an addict, I know all too well that being sedated comes at various prices, not the least of which is that whatever problem I was escaping, it was still there when the effect of the drug wore off. Sometimes it was even worse than before.

Neuroleptics are antipsychotic drugs that you might think are different because they are not tranquilizers. Wrong! Your first clue to being wrong is that this group of drugs is also known as major tranquilizers. What is particularly scary about this group is that they can produce Parkinson-like mental and physical side effects with the exception that the tremors (shakes) are not very evident. Those under the influence of this group of drugs are also described as having no interest, as being indifferent to what goes on around them, and as lacking concern for themselves and others. In short, they just vegetate while the world goes by. Sounds very similar to being stoned, does it not? It sounds especially familiar when I read that people under the influence of these prescribed drugs are not cured or relieved of their symptoms such as delusions or hearing voices. Under the influence, they just stop caring about them.

You should also know and be frightened by the main purpose behind prescribing neuroleptic drugs. The main reason is to subdue and control people who behave badly. This is accomplished by chemically and not physically (lobotomy) disabling the front part of the person's brain that makes us human. The part where we experience love, empathy, creativity, concern and care for others; the part that when destroyed makes robots out of us along with a bunch of other permanent distortions to our bodies and minds. A huge price, I think, for behaving badly. The only people I can imagine wanting to do this to another human being are the ones responsible for warehousing them in asylums, prisons or other secure, isolated, institutional settings. Docile people are easy to manage. Addressing their reasons for behaving badly takes time and energy; not that this reasoning makes it right, even in such institutions, let alone in the community.

I cannot stress enough therefore that before you consider taking such a prescribed drug or allowing it to be given to a loved one, especially a child you think long and hard before you agree to it. Most importantly, do the research, learn as much as you can. The information is out there just for the looking.

The fourth family of psychiatric drugs are mood stabilizers. Now, who among us would not want something at one time or another to stabilize our mood? Cut out the lows and highs and just sail along a gently rolling sea. By their name, this group of drugs sounds appealing. They especially sound appealing to those involved with people who unpredictably go between being very active doing all sorts of messed up things - to doing nothing for days, sometimes weeks or months. The questions by now are obvious: At what cost does this gently rolling sea come, and how is it achieved anyway?

You guessed it, mood stabilizing drugs also are sedatives. Not major, but minor ones, and the effect comes at a tremendous price, even a lethal one for some people. The most familiar of the mood stabilizer drugs is lithium. As I said, like cocaine, we were first introduced to it in a soda pop, specifically *7Up* and some brands of beer. It was believed to reduce uric acid in the body; the stuff that causes gout, your uncle's painful big toe. However, when it was proven not to dissolve uric acid crystals, the salt was not thrown out with the garbage because, when injected into guinea pigs, it made them docile. Not to waste this discovery, it was tried on humans with the desired effect of making them also docile; not as severely docile as neuroleptics make people, but still docile or sedated.

Not surprisingly, other mind-, cut people off from their feelings and from others because the drugs, too, are sedatives. Cut off in this way, ones motivation to do anything is hugely reduced. These are the emotional and behavioural costs to chemically sailing on gently rolling seas. The physical costs are memory loss and reduced in thinking abilities. These sedatives harm cells in the brain and the connections between them. The drugs also can harm organs like the kidneys. In fact, if not closely monitored through blood analyses, a drug like lithium can poison and eventually literally, as opposed to figuratively, kill a person.

If you are ever labelled as manic depressive, or as having a bipolar disorder, lithium is likely to be prescribed to subdue your manic (hyper) behaviour. Once you are subdued, there will be much effort put into convincing you to stay on it to prevent another manic episode. The harm of being on this sedating drug is far less, you will be told, than the harm you create during the manic phases of your way of coping with life. Not true, unless you are satisfied with having no life at all.

Lithium is not the only drug in this mind-altering family of chemicals. Interestingly, antiepileptic drugs also are used to stabilize mood swings. Because these drugs suppress, dampen or slow down electrical activity in the brain, you guessed it, they are also a form of sedative.

Some of you might say being sedated is not so bad, and some people should be sedated, if not forever, certainly for brief periods of time. I would have no problem agreeing, if not for the fact that almost always people are told that they must be on one or more sedative for the rest of their life. What they are not told is the devastating effect the drugs will have on their brain, organs, and body; damages that are not reversible. They are permanent, meaning for the rest of your life.

The last family of psychiatric drugs is stimulants. Stimulants, as many of you with street smarts know, are drugs like cocaine, amphetamines, nicotine, and caffeine, to name the best-known ones. By definition, they stimulate, jazz you up. Because of this effect, they also are used to 'treat' depression, stimulate appetite, and fight fatigue. Their current most popular use is with children who are labelled as having Attention Deficit Hyperactive Disorder (ADHD). Those of you who were raising children when using or when struggling through the initial phases of abstinence, probably had a run-in with this very popular label and how the establishment responds to it. So, it's important that you do your own research, but I will get you started here.

Just because so I read one in five American boys aged between 10 and 14 years, increasing numbers of girls, and now adults, are being prescribed a stimulant drug for ADHD, does not make it right. There are many reasons why it does not make it right, the most important being that the drug is used to suppress symptoms while the cause is ignored. While the way in which the symptoms are suppressed are harmful to children and adults, they are welcomed by teachers and significant others. The stimulant drugs are welcomed because they decrease activity and increase focus. They are harmful because the increased focus on a single task comes at the price of making the person completely unaware of everything else around them. As one mother shared with me, her son is so focused on crossing the street that he is completely unaware of the traffic around him that is going to run him down.

There are other prices to be paid for the focus on a single task. Ask children and adults lose interest in life, they become emotionally dull, and some behave like the zombies portrayed in those stupid movies. As you will recall from TWO, I was also prescribed Ritalin as a child. What I remember the most, is that it made me feel not like myself and prevented me from sleeping, which was my most effective way of escaping what I called my shit life.

The physical effects of stimulants also are very nasty. Children and adults can become addicted to them, and the physical growth of children can be obstructed by them. This can include the growth of the brain as well as other organs in the body.

As you can see, there are far more reasons for avoiding both prescribed and street stimulant drugs than for using them. The only understandable but unacceptable reason is that teachers like the way the drugs make troublesome children docile. For me, it is not a good enough reason. Hopefully, I have convinced you to think the same or, at the very least, to do your own research about stimulant drugs when the occasion requires it.

In summary, hopefully I have shown that prescribed drugs do not have 'condition-specific effects'. What this means is that antidepressants do not stop you from being depressed. Stimulants do not remove the reasons why a child is hyperactive; sleeping pills neither cure you of the reasons why you cannot sleep nor do they provide a restorative, sleep experience. Neuroleptic, antipsychotic drugs neither stop the voices nor the delusions through which desperate people escape their shit life, like I used to. Sedated, they just do not care. Mood stabilizers do in fact stabilize, as long as you don't mind being severely sedated and physically damaged for the rest of your life.

To conclude this long chapter, I want to say two important things. First, reading about this stuff is not easy and many of the people who write about the reality seem to beat around the bush. Often, they don't seem to want to get to the point. Perhaps, like in my small way here, they are being careful not to give the impression that the topic is simple. For me, for sure it was not, but the effort, because of what I learned, was well worth it. I urge you to do likewise. Spend the time, investigate and read as much as you can before you agree to take something that could harm or even kill you. Remember Mary's story.

Second, I want to repeat an important point I made earlier. No one person or group of people is to blame. Family physicians, psychiatrists, and some psychologists that prescribe these drugs really, truly believe they are helping. Most importantly, as I said before, they do not know what they do not know. That is why, in the USA, there have been successful lawsuits against the medical schools that produce biological psychiatrists. My understanding is that the schools are accused of being overly influenced by the drug companies that make the psychiatric drugs. The medical schools also are being held accountable for not letting the students know about all the stuff I read just because I am curious.

At the end of the day, I figure it all boils down to business, making the most amount of money with the least amount of effort. Drugging people is easier than problem solving with them fifty minutes at a time. If the effect of drugging is that they just don't care, and docile people are easier to be around than problematic ones, so much the better. At the very least, however, we should be properly informed about the kind of dance to which we are agreeing.

CHAPTER 8
Be Careful of the Establishment

This is a difficult chapter to write because most of me, almost all of me, believes no one is to blame for how much influence psychiatry has worldwide nor for its primary tool, drugs. Psychiatrists come by what they do through their education, conferences, in-service training, and the stuff they read after graduation. The drug companies, on the other hand, are something altogether different. Because they are corporations, their reason for existing is to make money, as much as they can, in any way they can. Their tactics include seducing medical schools and psychiatrists to do research and recommend the use of their drugs.

Our governments, so I read, are supposed to regulate and watch over what these drug manufacturers do. For example, they are supposed to make sure that they do not pollute the environment too much, that they don't conspire to fix prices that benefit them too much, and that their drugs do not harm us too much.

In theory, all this sounds good; in real life not so much. However, can you imagine in what shape the world would be if we had no regulations? Probably we would not be here at all. For the sake of profit, a long time ago, one or more companies would have poisoned or otherwise killed us all. So, thankfully we do have regulations that do some good.

Because of regulations, drugs cannot be just made and sold. There are complicated things that a pharmaceutical company has to do in order to be permitted to sell a drug. There is much written about the hoops they have to jump through and how sloppy the rules can get. What I found really interesting is that on virtually every psychiatric drug bottle or box there is a 'black box' that warns people about what harm the drug could cause. As mentioned before, the black box warns that an antidepressant could make depression worse, cause suicidal thoughts or even action, especially if prescribed to children. On other drugs, the black box warns that the chemical could cause or make worse anxiety, agitation, panic attacks, insomnia, irritability, hostility, impulsivity, and the list goes on. I can't help but think Mary probably was prescribed this drug or something like it.

Then there are warnings about stopping a drug suddenly, because that, too, could make a person feel worse, even do something completely out of character.

Since there are black box warnings for all psychiatric drugs to speak of, people being uninformed about the dangers of taking them is a very curious thing. On the other one hand, people may not be told of the black box warning. The may be told only about some but not all of the dangers. On the other hand, they may be told but they do not care or hear only what I heard, "this will make you feel better".

At some level, I believe, all addicts know that taking something to "feel better" is a drug regardless of who is selling it. Because the feel-good stuff is a drug, when we stop taking it, there are consequences. Mostly the 'feeling good', which is being sedated until you do not care, stops and reality comes out of hiding. That is why addicted addicts use daily until they are fed up with their chemically-created, unreal life. When I started on my abstinence and reality came out of hiding, I naively expected that the establishment would have answers that would not harm me. Wrong! But what about the people with mental or behavioural problems who are not addicted addicts or addicted? How could they be so naïve not to ask about side effects or the dangers of taking psychiatrist- prescribed drugs? The only answer that makes sense to me is that, for no real good reason, they trust the establishment because they are part of it or are perspiring to be. Pretty dangerous behaviour, if you ask me, especially if you bring your child into this nasty dance hall.

Unfortunately, this is exactly what parents do worldwide every day. I have seen it with my own eyes. Schools and child welfare agencies require the parents of a troubled child to get "that child treated". Almost always, the treatment includes some stimulant-drug like Ritalin. Parents are told it is a responsible thing to do and, at the same time, are warned that if they do not act as responsible parents and drug their child, the child will be considered at risk and will be taken from them. How this all came to be is quite amazing. My best 'informed' guess, is that there are two reasons why all this happened.

The first reason is that few, if any, parents want (are able) to take responsibility for screwing up their child. My parents did not. They blamed my teachers and me for being an 'idiot', a name they called me many times. Second, and a little more complex reason, it is easier to accept that the person 'caught' a mental illness from, let's say a doorknob, than to accept responsibility for inadequate parenting and creating a horrible environment for a child. I have heard parents say the kid's behaviour has nothing to do with home life or the environment, since the child has a medical condition and is being medicated for it.

If parents hate to admit that they screwed up their children, what about the community, society or culture in which parents do it? What leader, elected politician, parish priest, minister, rabbi, or educator would want to admit that the environment over which they have influence, some even control, are conditions for the creation of addicts and various forms of madness. No one, I think. They would all rather blame it on some disease or genetics which they do not understand but, at some level, recognize as a very convenient way of escaping responsibility for creating it.

After yet another mass shooting, I saw President Trump doing a "fancy dance" to blame something else than the ease with which guns can be obtained in the USA. He was blaming the shooting on the person's "mental health problem". That is correct, I thought, but he does not realize to what he is admitting. From everything I read and learned in a very short time, I was able to figure out that he was admitting to staggering social problems in the great USA; social problems that are increasing in number and severity. We see troubled people murdering many for some legal or illegal drug that probably caused their bizarre reasoning.

What you never hear about, as I said before, is the 'treatment' the so-called mentally ill were receiving. You also never hear about what prescribed drug they were being treated with. As we know by now, just by reading this far, many drugs prescribed by psychiatrists can cause worsening of symptoms and violent, aggressive as well as suicidal behaviours. I think it would be very interesting if someone investigated these acts of horrible violence to find out if the offender was seeing a psychiatrist and what prescribed drug or drugs the person was taking. That would be a very threatening study.

Because of the threat, such a study is not likely to be funded or supported. At some level, most people know that the results just might destroy a convenient way out of taking personal, community, and social responsibility for the messed up people we create, me being a good example. Instead of blaming bad behaviour on an illness or disease, we just might have to look at ourselves in the mirror and take responsibility for what we have done. At least for now I cannot imagine anyone willing to do this. Therefore, I don't think such a study will be conducted in the foreseeable future.

I need now to warn those of you who might decide, after reading all of this, to go off your psychiatrist-prescribed drugs. Don't do it! I repeat, do not do it. It is not that easy. It is as difficult as it was for you addicted addicts to go off street drugs or alcohol. Most of you, and me, did it in a detox. You need the same kind of help with prescribed drugs. Good luck with finding such help. According to my friends, physicians are not too eager to get involved. You just might have to settle and check into a regular detox center once again. So much more reason for not getting started with this legal, establishment-drug industry in the first place, especially after you already kicked the street-drug industry to the curb.

CHAPTER 9
Fix Both the Symptom and the Problem

I n this chapter, I will try to explain some important differences based on my experiences. The first on my list is the difference between a symptom, like anxiety, and what's causing it. The second on my list is the difference between suppressing, quieting down, dampening or turning down the volume of a symptom and fixing it. I already talked about symptoms being warning signs of something serious going on. Both have to be fixed, often first the symptom and then the cause. Fixing almost always never means being cured or making something troublesome go away. Mostly, it means getting it under control or learning to live with it.

The psychiatric solution almost always focuses on suppressing a symptom like anxiety by sedating you; sometimes, sedating you to the point that you don't care about the symptom or for that fact, anything else. While getting sedated like that might sound appealing, getting and being sedated can come at a significant cost. Also, just because a prescribed drug can make you feel better, what is called "medication spellbound," that does not mean the problem causing it is gone. Every addicted addict and every addicted person who has escaped unpleasantness through a "high" knows this. The difference is that illegal drug users sometimes do sober up, whereas the psychiatric plan is mostly to keep you sedated indefinitely. That means for the rest of your life. Do not forget the price at which "forever sedated" comes. If you chose this path for you or a loved one, just do it with eyes wide open.

If you chose a different path, a path like I chose and the one that Mary never had a chance to choose, some getting in touch with reality is required. This starts with releasing your obstructed developmental potential, growing up. If you can learn to cope with not having a pot-bellied stove, you can also learn to get under control or better manage anxiety, panic attacks, fear, sadness and even being always aggressive to protect yourself from real or imagined threats to your very life.

All that is required is a great deal of hard work. Is that all?" You might ask. The answer is a yes, with a qualified, it is worth it!

The challenge is knowing what the work is and finding the right person to help the work get done. Most often, and this is worth repeating, the work has less to do with symptoms than with causes. At first, my stubborn focus was on the symptoms. That is why I got sucked in by the psychiatric "this will make you feel better" promise. Thankfully, I found the right counsellor to get me focused on what really matters: the cause of my symptoms.

The first work that had to be done was getting to know and believe that a symptom like anxiety or a panic attack is not going to kill me. The second work that had to be done was to understand that most, if not all, of my symptoms were caused by the very real emotion, fear. From the very beginning of my life, starting in the womb, I had real good reasons to be afraid, often to fear for my very life. This always triggered the stress-reaction hormone, cortisol. Its constant presence and the absence of empathic nurturance, both of which I explained before, prevented me from building that critically important pot-bellied stove in the womb and during the first two years of my life.

No wonder fear has been a constant companion all my life. And I came by it for good reasons. Coping with it involved running (getting stoned) or barking loudly, like a terrified dog to scare off a possible attacker. Of course, this kind of life made me very sad.

So, you see, from doing good, guided work, I was able to understand that the cause of my negative emotions was not some imbalance of chemicals or nerves breaking down. My symptoms were caused by real, horrible, life experiences, experiences which could not be undone.

If the experiences did not affect me in a negative way now, that would be really weird. So, I concluded, those negative emotions were appropriate responses to the shit life I had until I decided to get and stay abstinent. If sedating me without my informed consent to the point my emotions did not bother me was my only choice, I might as well have stayed on street drugs or continued to get drunk every day. Not the choice I made.

The challenge at this phase in my journey was to figure out how to stop or not to feel so bad, when the reason for doing so was long gone. I had to learn and accept that as a sober, competent adult, I no longer had to fear for my life and have the symptoms of anxiety, panic attacks, and all the rest. Getting the cause under control also brought the roar of the symptoms down to a dull, barely able- to-hear noise.

Getting to this point was not easy and I needed help. Certainly not prescription drugs but what, I did not know at the start. The first, on the top of the establishment list, I ruled out but not before scaring myself, especially seeing Mary die in that horrible way. But finding alternative help was very difficult because of cost. Establishment-biological-psychiatrist fees are covered in Canada by our comprehensive healthcare plan. In other countries, psychiatric services are the first to be paid by various insurance plans. Even though not all psychiatrists rely primarily on drugs to make people "feel better", based on my experience, good luck finding one who will take the time to get to know you and has the skills to help you cope in better ways other than getting stoned.

I had some very difficult choices to make. One, having to choose a counsellor. The other deciding what counselling approach would help me the most. As you can imagine, there are many approaches to choose from, almost as many as the counsellors who provide them. My method for choosing involved looking at the beliefs of the various disciplines as I described above. But I must admit, having been burned once, my focus was more on the person than on the approach the counsellor used. Later I learned this was the best strategy. As you probably guessed, I chose a social worker to guide me through this part of my journey.

My work began, and it's worth repeating, with understanding and accepting that there is no cure for me being me. But from understanding who I am, I began to slowly discover, much good can come of it. The good being learning to control my emotions (symptoms) and what was causing them. It was helpful to think especially of the causes as demons – sinister, tricky, vile creatures always lurking in the shadows ready and able to mess me up whenever the opportunity presented itself. Realizing this, I accepted personal responsibility to be on my guard for the rest of my life, just to keep them under control.

Demons or other vile creatures in horror movies are scary mostly because they are in the shadows and you only see glimpses of them. In order to take away the power of my demons over me, I had to shine a bright light on them and then examine them from every angle over a long period of time. Let me tell you, this really worked. However, while this level of understanding was necessary, it was not enough. I had to do a lot of work to make it real. The work involved a great deal of reading and a growing ability to talk honestly about everything. This leaving out the bullshit was like releasing me from an awful prison. The saying, the truth will set you free, became a very real and pleasant discovery.

I am raving about my positive experiences with counselling because I am comparing it to my very nasty, almost deadly experience with psychiatry. But I do know that talk therapy, counselling, is not without its critics. I also know that there is not one sure-fire approach to counselling and, as a result, many people are down on it. But I also know, from personal experience, that what really matters in talk therapy is the person you are talking with. Once you establish that the person has the credentials and license to do therapy, the next big question to be answered is your compatibility, how you think you are going to get along with him or her. While there are many ways of figuring this out, I think there are some basic things to consider. To start, see if you find the person likable because you believe the person listens, wants to get to know you, is genuinely curious about you, accepts your reactions to experiences as real and justifiable and above all seems to know a lot more about how to live life better than you do.

I want to share two examples of how knowing that we are all a product of our early environment and, as a result, we all have demons, works. The first example is my lifelong constant emotion of fear, a symptom of how I was raised. As I described in *TWO*, the parenting I received during the first two years of life was so horrible that at times I was in real danger of dying, even being killed. While hard to accept, it was true. However, as a street-smart abstinent adult, I was no longer vulnerable, but still afraid. In fact, my street smarts and experiences made me into a pretty tough person, much harder to kill than an infant. Therefore, my early, life-learned fear of all things was no longer a justifiable reaction as an adult. The evaluation of most situations as dangerous, as a capable adult, became the demon to be understood and controlled. It took some time, and I am still working on it, probably for the rest of my life but I'm getting there.

The next example is my demon that causes me constant anxiety. The demon comes from missed opportunities to learn or acquire a sense of confidence to manage whatever life brings my way each and every day. Without the confidence that is learned by successfully dealing with crap when it comes along, I was justifiably anxious all the time, sometimes to be panicked by virtually almost nothing. To bring this examined-in-the-light-of-honesty demon under control, I had to respond to its irrationality with rational facts about how many times and how well I had successfully dealt with things, including crap, getting and staying sober or, as I now like to call it, abstinent from all intoxicants. Again, I am still working on it, but I'm getting there.

I hope these brief examples will encourage you to get help to identify and get to know your demons, because from knowing and understanding them comes the ability to get these lifelong companions under control. Sober, growing-up addicts are great examples of the benefits of so doing.

So, I ask you again, is this not a better way of getting your troublesome emotions and messed-up behaviours under control than fixing some chemical imbalance that cannot be seen or measured, or, even worse, fixing the imaginary imbalance with a sedative that comes with harmful side effects, until you no longer care about how you feel, think or behave?

I want to conclude in this final chapter with another, strong warning: there are no fixes or cures for who we are, let alone easy ones. Searching for one is foolish, dangerous or can even cost you your life. Honour Mary by remembering her story and by learning from it. Hopefully, the benefit of writing this third book is that you will never be in the position to say: "No one told me".

Last but not least, please do not, I repeat, do not just take my word for it. There are many scholarly books out there with the same information and warning. The books provide many examples of what can go wrong in the search for a quick and easy, establishment-approved fix. If you read one book about this topic, I guarantee your outrage will motivate you to read others. You will then become part of the solution, instead of the problem, and will find purpose and meaning to your life. Mine is to spread the word and try to save others from having to experience what Mary and I had to endure.

REFLECTIONS

Introduction

Not as a disclaimer but in the interest of transparency, I want to make it perfectly clear that I am primarily a messenger about psychiatry and the harm the discipline perpetrates with its prescribed drugs. I wish I were not. I wish I had been better informed decades before and had taken better care to know more about what many of my clients had to endure while dancing with psychiatry. Initially, as a new graduate, I accepted the establishment-awarded status of psychiatry as well as the publicized benefits of their various magical potions. In my defense, there was some but certainly not enough critical information about psychiatry in my graduate education. I did, however, know about the ideas of Thomas Szasz and R.D. Lang. While I read and referenced them, unfortunately, I did not engage in sufficiently meaningful discussions about their message. Moreover, it was not until recently, a decade or more, that I became aware that both Sigmund Freud and Carl Jung raised the alarm about the dangers of the emerging new discipline of psychiatry and its collaborative partnership with the psycho-pharmaceutical industry.

Sadly, to really get my attention about this topic, it took

a catastrophe - the death of a close friend in the so-called care of a psychiatrist. It took some time, but I am now committed to joining the ranks of many others to spread the word. My primary goal in writing this third book of four in the trilogy is to mobilize your curiosity to read at least one of the references provided in this book. Once you become better informed, hopefully you will join the ranks of those who shun exchanging illegal intoxicants for prescribed ones. Most importantly, I hope you will think long and hard before choosing a specialist in psychiatry to help you or a loved one cope with the difficulty that is life.

Now, for the obligatory and genuine warning:

Most psychiatric drugs are powerful intoxicants. They can and do cause havoc on your body and mind, especially if you decide to abruptly stop taking them. Do not make things worse than they already are. Seek a professional's help, one that has the relevant expertise. You might have to check yourself into a detox facility when coming off a prescribed drug, regardless of what it is and how strong the dose is.

I am compelled to end this introduction to reflections by admitting that I believe psychiatric drugs (sedatives especially) have a purpose, albeit a limited one in some circumstances for some people. For example, I was glad my mother was prescribed, for a limited time, a sedative when she was so distraught about the death of my father. I am also glad that there is sedation for some of my completely out-of-control forensic clients. In fact, for a particularly violent man, I recommended and advocated his sedation. However, my recommendation was to prescribe him marijuana, which he preferred and would faithfully consume rather than the psychiatric drug that made him feel "weird". Age and life stages have taught me to avoid absolutes whenever possible, even about psychiatry and their drugs.

"Better" is a Relative Term

We often talk of "better" without giving much thought to what we mean by it. The optician, in determining what corrective glasses are needed, asks, "better or worse?" when changing the test lenses. It is one of the few times "better" is the appropriate concept to use. When it is "better", the image on the eye chart is clear and you can make out the letters easily. In most other situations, the appropriate descriptor is "different". This includes comparing the life of being a stoner to being abstinent. The temptation is to call abstinence, especially in the beginning, better. In reality, it is just different. Being new to abstinence comes with its own challenges which can be quite a surprise, as it was for Sally and Mary, and as I witnessed with almost all my clients transitioning from one state of being to another. Often, the unpleasantly surprised persons give up and go back to their previous life that includes remaining cognitive developmentally stuck. Some, like Sally and Mary, try a path of least resistance. They try the quick, easy fix of psychiatric drugs which is nothing more than an orchestrated myth. Hard to blame them though, who could resist being seduced by a promise of an easy fix? But as we have seen, being "medication spellbound" (Breggin, 2008) does not last before the mind-altering prescription drugs start to take their toll.

Given these realities, I have always exercised great caution about the words I use with clients. My objective is to ensure their expectations are realistic, especially as they transition from being stoned to being abstinent, and from being cognitive developmentally stuck to getting unstuck. Initially, better is hardly a realistic expectation. Different is the initial result that becomes "better" when cognitive growth starts to emerge. For a myriad of reasons, life for the cognitive developmentally actualised is always better and easier. Decisions lead to sustainable, meaningful outcomes. Life becomes predictable, and accumulative gains are the norm as opposed to the exception. Most importantly, this state represents living in harmony with our nature as life-long evolving beings, not stuck ones.

Activating our cognitive, developmental potential takes a great deal of work that is well worth it. The best example is the benefits of reaching that stage at which the creation of pleasing fantasies is no longer easy and the person is able to say, "I have a very serious problem". This then leads to "different", which then becomes "better".

Emotions Released

Since virtually all of us have endured some trauma during our formative and early years, for certain there are troublesome emotions (demons) lurking in the crevasses of our minds. This lurking some refer to as suppressed or subconscious emotions. Regardless, they are there for all of us, just waiting for an opening to reveal themselves and compromise the quality of our lives. The opening for addicted addicts and those addicted is when they first achieve abstinence. When they become abstinent for a while, it is like taking a heavy, wet blanket off smouldering ambers. Once the air gets to them, all of a sudden, there is a surprising raging fire. "Where did this come from?" is quickly followed by, "put it out right now". How, does not matter. All that matters is to extinguish the blaze.

Being in this state makes people like Sally and Mary extremely vulnerable. Their lack of experience and knowledge about psychiatry and its drugs also makes them victims. Consenting without realizing that they are consenting - let alone understanding to what they have consented filling the prescription and taking the first pill, all meet the criteria of a duped victim.

The analogy of a raging fire, I believe, accurately reflects the intensity of the negative emotions and that these emotions are closely related. To give them separate labels begs the question: for what purpose? (unless the purpose is to prescribe a pill for each one, which a distraught person like Sally does not need nor will benefit from).

What the person needs is validation that their feelings (negative emotions) are caused by real current and past experiences, and that it is logically consistent that they are sad about all of it. Instead of medicating - more accurately sedating - the individual, the responsible and morally principled reaction is to learn to control the conditions (demons) responsible for creating the negative emotions

Willful Blindness or Something Else

At one time or another, we have all been willfully blind to something; sometimes, wilfully blind about a person, sometimes an activity, and sometimes ourselves. Looking for quick fixes could be willful blindness about the reality that, almost always, there is no such thing. Sally's experience and how she tells it beg a different explanation. Her need for a quick fix of her emotional problems when abstinent was child-like. Children do not have the fully developed ability to postpone gratification; they want what they want, when they want it – not later, but now. And they want it through the path of least resistance. Developmentally stuck adults behave the same way. Sally, just at the onset of her starting to grow up, was still mostly disposed to creating pleasing fantasies or to being seduced by them.

Similarly, most election campaign strategies pander to the electorate's cognitive, developmental propensity to be seduced by pleasing fantasies. The discipline of psychiatry and its life partner, the psycho-pharmaceutical industry (not to be outdone by politicians), have embraced the same strategy and have greatly benefited from it. In fact, the two have become the most successful imperialistic organizations of all time. The two have intentionally created new markets and have globally infiltrated every nook and cranny of this world. While their market strategies are laudable (Davies, 2013), their success probably is more attributable to the promise of a quick, easy fix and to the appeal the medical model has because it allows for the abdication of familial, community, and social responsibility for creating badly behaved children (addicts), who then become badly behaved adults (addicted addicts).

The imperialistic success of the psycho-pharmaceutical industry and especially of biological psychiatry is their appeal, and their appeal reveals a great deal about the cognitive developmental status of people everywhere. Based on the success of the two partners, it would not be unreasonable to advance the premise that more people are cognitive developmentally stuck than not. Therefore, the majority of people are quite easily seduced by pleasing fantasies of a quick, easy fix, and that they are not responsible for the mess the world is in.

This same premise can easily be advanced about psychiatry. As noted earlier, the pharmaceutical industry, however, is a whole other story. To be sure, there are some seriously scholarly dissenters to the biological model among the ranks of psychiatry. The significant ones are referenced in this book. But for the most part, the majority of practitioners buy into their discipline's belief systems (Whitaker & Cosgrove, 2015). As their unwitting patients, they also behave as cognitive developmentally stuck, prone to creating and to being seduced by pleasing fantasies of easy and quick fixes to the problems of living. On the other hand, perhaps not. Perhaps it is all about the mother of all sins, greed (Tickle,

2004). The preferred, more palatable explanation for me is the cognitive developmentally stuck one.

Let me illustrate by way of an example. As I was writing this reflections section, a friend well-entrenched in the establishment, loaned me a book written by two biological psychiatrists. He introduced the authors (Goldbloom and Bryden, 2016) as the "real thing". True to the introduction they certainly are. Both are clearly the real product of intense socialization into the values, beliefs and behaviours of their chosen discipline. They genuinely believe in the reliability and validity of their diagnostic manual (DSM5) and the benefits of drugs they prescribe. Not surprisingly, they even praise the practice of electroconvulsive therapy (ECT). To their credit, they do not discount the benefits of talk therapy but see it mostly as an adjunct to their psycho-pharmaceutical intervention. They also acknowledge the ambiguities in making a diagnosis but, nevertheless, resort to prescribing, hopefully in the interest of at least "calming" symptoms, an intention that is never clearly articulated.

The authors are truly representative of how one becomes a "real thing", biological psychiatrist. It takes much socialization and drinking of the *Kool-Aid* being served by the group to which they are clearly committed to belong. While genuinely caring and intent on helping those in need, they are, without knowing, cognitive developmentally stuck at the reference group, tribal perspective.

Involuntary Intoxication and All That Comes With It

There is a great deal written about what harm is done by psychiatric drugs. Peter Breggin, a psychiatrist who has not drunk the Kool-Aid is probably the most eminent among the authors but there are many others. I have provided a sampling of them with the hope that reading one will whet your appetite to read more.

To get you started, let's first look at the absence of informed consent. It is exactly what it sounds like. You are given insufficient, if any at all, information about what the prescribed pill will do to you. Since the primary effect is to alter the state of your mind, it is referred to as "involuntary intoxication". What happens next is called "medication spellbinding". This means that the people taking a prescribed drug have very little, if any, awareness as to what effect the drug is having on their brain function. Most are virtually unaware of how bizarre their ideas have become, and in that state can commit way-out-of character actions. For this very reason, the investigation of bizarre, sometimes murderous, actions of people with so called 'mental illness' should include information about what psychiatric drug(s) they just started taking, have been taking, or just stopped taking. Sadly, this is seldom done unless a malpractice law suit is initiated by the significant others of the acting out-of-character perpetrator and/or victim(s). In the legal realm, there are many case studies including action taken against the schools from which the psychiatrist graduated. Rightfully, the reasoning is that the graduate only knows what was in the curriculum, which incidentally is significantly influenced by drug manufacturers.

Next in getting you started, is information about the myriad of side effects produced by psychiatric drugs. Some alter the physiology of the brain, which causes chain reaction conditions, the names of which all start with 'tardive'. The word means, caused by medication. By way of examples, here are some drug-induced conditions: potentially lethal diabetes, pancreatitis, fever, global mental disruption, disfiguring grimaces, tics and abnormal body movements that can be permanent. These are just a sampling of side effects, that you too, as Sally, could easily find out just by looking.

You may be shocked to learn that electroshock therapy (ECT) continues to be practiced to this day. It is an archaic assault on the brain similar to blasting your car engine with a shotgun when it is not running well. The shock causes disorientation, confusion, memory loss, sometimes to the extent of erasing all memory. These and more severe damage to the brain often are permanent, not unlike the surgical removal of parts of the brain, otherwise known as a lobotomy. While this is no longer performed (hopefully), sadly assaulting the brain chemically and electrically continues.

If you are in any way starting to or are already involved in this dangerous system, do your own research before it is too late. If you are already spellbound, hopefully a significant other will advocate on your behalf and/or organize an intervention.

Operational Definitions and Outcome Measures

There are two major themes in chapter 4: one concerns the need to generate operational (measurable and observable) definitions; the other concerns, to what we attribute strange/unusual behaviour.

Operationally, defining 'better', you may agree, is not an easy task. Perhaps, this is why the concept "better" is used, and why few think to ask what it means.

The next theme, why Sally is not feeling so good, concerns the cause of it. Throughout the ages, some have considered strange behaviour, madness, to be an illness. Others considered it to be simply bad behaviour caused by social/environmental conditions. Arguably, the currently predominant, most popular view is that most strange behaviours came from a biological illness. The fact that no genetic or organic causes have been found for all but less than ten conditions, is lost on both the practitioner and the victims of their services.

Medicalizing behavioural and emotional problems is very discouraging. While there is a current call for increased focus on "mental health" this, too, is discouraging because the call invariably translates into a need for more psychiatrists and more services from them. I wrote about this (Polgar, 2019) to alert other counselling professionals I argued that this is no longer a trend. It is now an entrenched reality; a genie that will be very difficult to stuff back into the proverbial bottle. Perhaps the successful lawsuits for aggressively marketing opioids just might encourage those harmed by psychiatry to do the same.

It is already happening. Angry survivors of involuntary intoxication and medically-caused brain damage are challenging the authority, prestige and influence of psychiatry. Eventually, as we all become fully informed, we can then channel our energies in to prevention through deliberate strategies designed to create environments conducive to the actualization of the human, developmental potential (Polgar, 2011).

Words Matter

For a long time now, I have had a problem with the phrases "mental health" and "Alcoholics Anonymous". The concept "health" bothers me when used in conjunction with "mental". The problem, as I see it, is that the word, health, conjures up something physical. Therefore, the implication is that something physical is causing the mental problem. Add to this the concepts of "illness" and "disease", the conclusion that there is a medical problem is ensured, which is in the realm of a medical professional to address. The use of these words in the context of mental also conjures up unrealistic expectations of a cure. Not unrealistic, if indeed there is a physical problem, since we do get cured from illnesses caused by external organisms or internal functions going awry. However, since there is no organic basis for almost all "mental illnesses", an expectation of being cured is, to say the least, unrealistic. Being an addict optimally illustrates this point.

It is also noteworthy that psychiatry in its almost thousand-page manual (DSM5) talks of *disorders*, not illnesses or diseases.

We therefore need to invent a phrase more appropriate

and relevant to the problem; a phrase that will invoke different thinking and different actions. 'Dysfunctional' is a familiar concept to counsellors from the various disciplines, as is 'maladaptive'. Add to this the role environment and relationships play in how we function, the term "psychosocially dysfunctional", while a mouthful, is a good place to start breaking down the medical monopoly we have unwittingly allowed to take root.

The focus on alcohol is long past the relevance it had in the 1940s. The proliferation of various intoxicating drugs and their availability was just emerging. Alcohol was the most readily available substance to which addicts became addicted. This is no longer the case. Also, on close examination, to what substance addicts become addicted is of little relevance to how a 12-step based program works. Given these current realities, Addicts Anonymous would be an appropriate name change. Thankfully, in an increasing number of locations, the focus on alcohol has been replaced by a focus on being an addict. While a slow process, the fact that it is happening is encouraging. But tribalism, even in 12-step programs, is alive and well. The avoidable problems this creates is the impetus for making this trilogy about addiction into a four-book exercise.

The Quest for a Biological Cause Stubbornly Persists

As this was being written, The Atlantic periodical publication enthusiastically reported about a "landmark" study on the origins of alcoholism. The enthusiasm was based on an evolving, biological explanation and a possible biological fix in pill form. Good news indeed. Who among us would not welcome an easy, quick fix for this life-compromising condition? And who among us would not cherish being that hero in shining armour providing it? Well, the biological psychiatrist doing the study is "perspiring" to be just that person.

The researcher is described in the article as a seasoned psychiatrist. True to his socialization into the discipline, he is seeking the holy grail of a biological cause for alcoholism, out of which will come a biological cures, of course, after more research, probably at least five more years. Not an unfamiliar refrain especially concerning things in need of a biological fix waiting for that promising cure for male pattern baldness announced way over five years ago.

We are told in The Atlantic, that the research psychiatrist

is not alone in the quest for a cure for alcoholism. A French cardiologist claims to have cured himself of alcoholism by taking the drug Baclofen. Others claim similar success by taking benzodiazepins. What they fail to report, is that the drugs come with their own baggage, not the least of which is the ease with which people build up tolerance to them, an effect that sounds very much like becoming addicted to them instead of alcohol. Pick your poison, I guess.

What the physician-specialist in psychiatry is saying to be the biological basis, indeed the genetic cause of alcoholism, is the role of the chemical GABA in the amygdale of the brain. Without getting too heavily into the reeds of the alleged biochemical processes, the physician-researchers report that low activity of the GABA chemical in a rat's brain impairs the animal's ability to cope with fear and stress. This conclusion is based on the observed preference of such rats for alcohol, even when it is made to taste not so good. The logic of the experiment methodology and conclusion is at best questionable.

Less than stellar research design and formulations could be tolerated if not for the harm created by the false hope being advanced. The harm comes in the unintended discrediting of psychosocial explanations and concomitant interventions. Without realising or intending these researchers are purveyors of false hope of the worst kind and we will probably never hear from them again, let alone in five years. But they, and The Atlantic reporting about their work at the very least diminish the relevance of the psychosocial model and curtail the progress that comes from it, as for example, distinguishing between being an addicted addict and being addicted. To even talk about alcoholism now as if it is a real thing, as opposed to an addict who prefers alcohol, is conceptually regressive. It serves no other purpose than to bolster the public image of biological psychiatry that there is a genetic physical cause for this particular dysfunctionality.

In their eagerness to find a biological cause for alcoholism, the psychiatrists are missing an important discovery. Their discovery is not explaining why people abuse alcohol, rather it is probably explaining the underlying biology to the different temperaments with which human, dogs, cats, koi fish, parrots – all creatures, big and small – are born. Perhaps the biological psychiatrist and his colleagues have discovered the physical basis for being a 'highly sensitive person', a disposition first identified two decades ago (Aron, 1996). Perhaps, if the researchers read this, they will shift their focus to 'curing' highly sensitive people with a pill. Horrors. What will be next? Chemically homogenizing the temperament of all creatures?

In TWO (Polgar, 2019), I recommended that we treat all our newborns throughout their formative years and long after as if they were all highly sensitive. Then, they will receive the empathic nurturance they need to prevent all sorts of later life negative consequences, including being made an addict. Sally, Mary, and many other addicted addicts and dysfunctional adults probably start out in life as highly sensitive people, a way of being that has many benefits, once understood and harnessed.

Study Ties the Gut To Depression: and the Quest Goes On and On

J ust when I thought I was finished with this third book of four, my local newspaper on October 7, 2019, published yet another promising new approach to treating depression. Researchers at McMaster University's Brain Body Institute published in Scientific Reports that a common class of antidepressants 'work' (not defined) by stimulating activity in the gut, rather than in the brain, as previously believed. This, according to the researchers, "hints" at new treatment possibilities for depression; no doubt, possibilities in pill form. Of course, the possibilities are said to be in the future. No time estimates are given.

In the research report, the authors state that previously certain antidepressant drugs were believed to have worked (ie. cured depression?) by adjusting serotonin levels in the brain. But since 90 percent of serotonin is now believed to be produced in the gut, researchers hope that stimulating the vagus nerve of the gut will be an effective treatment for depression. This is yet another example of the persistent search for a biological cause and a biological chemical cure for it.

To say the very least, the quest of biological psychiatry and its ever-involved partner, the psycho-pharmaceutical industry, is alive and well. One has to admire their tenacious persistence.

After this brief admiration of their tenacity, we have to get real and once again examine what is being claimed. The first and most important point is that no drug actually treats depression or, for that matter, almost all other psychiatric disorders. The drugs sedate people to the point that they stop caring about what real life circumstances are causing them to be sad, depressed, anxious, panicky – and the list goes on and on. Second, and of equal importance, there are no physiological markers for depression. No blood analysis or imaging is used to diagnose a person as depressed, or almost all of the other disorders described in that thousand-page DSM5. If there is a biochemical imbalance, it is caused by psychiatric drugs. No surprise, since the drugs are developed precisely for the purpose of causing chemical imbalances (Breggin, 2008).

The purveying of false hope for a quick, easy fix, along with the opportunity to abdicate responsibility, continues. It is an attractive message, especially for the cognitive developmentally stuck, who also happen to be the creators of adverse environments in which addicts are created and from which many layers of psychosocial dysfunctionalities come.

Sadly, experience teaches that the McMaster researchers will never recant their promising, biological hope. Not one will exclaim, "what was I thinking?". They will persist, because it is how they were socialised and, as a result, what they believe. Targeting them with alternative information is of little benefit. So, the target has to be people like Sally, without a vested interest or bias; people who are genuinely curious and eager to understand, especially after an avoidably tragic loss like Mary; people who are willing to do the hard but surmountable work of learning to manage the demons life has given them.

No Free Lunches

To quote the Dalai Lama, "life is difficult". Why this idea is hard to accept, and why most rail against this reality is a profound marker of obstructed cognitive developmental potential. The adolescent mind seeks perfection and creates pleasing fantasies as to what it looks like. Consistent with the stage specific, cognitive perspective of living by pleasing fantasies, they also believe themselves to be entitled to it (Polgar, 2011). Sadly, this applies not only to the chronologically young, but also to the chronologically old-but-stuck majority. And we all pay a price for this reality, sometimes with our lives.

People like Sally, Mary, and all others enamoured with the promises of psychiatry, need to 'grow up', unleash their cognitive developmental potential, and face the reality that life is difficult, and then get on with keeping the difficulty down to a dull roar. Address the reasons for being anxious, panicky, depressed, wanting to escape into a fantasy of self-created reality and all the disorders listed in that almost thousand-page DSM5 psychiatric manual. There is no cure for how we have been shaped by life experiences but with effort and guidance, we can sure improve the quality of our lives in spite of it being difficult. I have seen hundreds of Sallies do it, and their successes make the avoidable deaths of the Maries and the suicides of medicated children that much more intolerable.

Instead of looking for that proverbial free lunch, an easy, quick fix, we all need to do the work. Even the slightest success will empower you to continue working on activating the potential with which we were all born.

Please challenge, if you can, my data based formulation that the impirialistic success and broad popularity of psychiatry is attributable to the cognitive developmentally obstructed predisposition of the majority to seek immediate relief from mental and emotional distress. The relief for most is temporary and eventually comes at a price. If your experience with prescribed intoxicants has been different, explaining and sharing why would be a great benefit to all those who continue to be or are about to be harmed.

REFERENCES

Aron, E.N. (1996). *The highly sensitive person: How to thrive when the world overwhelms you*. New York, NY: Harmony Press.

Aron was among the first to identify the phenomenon of this personality type. I believe there are far more people like this than we realize, and the information in the book can be very useful for self-awareness, as well as understanding people.

Breggin, P. (2008). *Medication madness: The role of psychiatric drugs in cases of violence, suicide and crime.* New York, NY: St. Martin's Press.

A pioneer in recognizing the dangers of psychiatry and their drugs, this book cites example after case example of what can go very wrong.

Davies, J. (2013). *Cracked: Why psychiatry is doing more harm than good.* London, UK: Icon Books Ltd.

Davies is a medical and social anthropologist. While this book is scholarly, it is an easy read. Probably, it should be the first book you read on this topic.

Frankl, Victor, E. (1959*). **Man's search for meaning.** Boston: Beacon Press.

Everyone should read this short book, it has a powerful message. It is especially recommended to the recently abstinent, freed from intoxicants and in search of new meaning and purpose to their life.

Goldbloom, D. & Bryden, P. (2016). ***How can I help? A week in my life as a psychiatrist.*** New York: Simon and Schuster.

I include this reference for two reasons. The book is a great example of biological psychiatrists' genuine beliefs, values and intervention strategies. The authors are the products of a lengthy and rigorous socialization process to the group they choose to belong. I also want to demonstrate that I am very much aware of the other side of the coin.

McVey Neufeld, K.A., Bienenstock, J., Bharwani, A., Champagne-Jorgensen, K., Mao, Y.K., West, C., Liu, Y., Kunze, W., & Forsythe, P. (2019). Oral selective serotonin reuptake inhibitors activate vagus nerve dependant gut-brain signalling. **Scientific Reports,** 9, 14290. https://doi.org/10.1038/s41598-019-50807-8

This is just one of many examples of the zeal with which research dollars are spent on justifying the beliefs and tactics of biological psychiatry.

Moncrieff, J. (2008). ***The myth of the chemical cure: A critique of psychiatric drug treatment.*** New York, NY: Palgrave McMillan. Basingstoke.

Moncrieff is a psychiatrist who understands chemistry and what drugs do to the body and mind. Her book is a challenge to read, but if you want to really dig down into the mythology of a chemical cure, this is the book to read.

Polgar, A.T. (2002). ***Because we can we must: Achieving the human developmental potential in five generations.*** Hamilton, ON: Sandriam Publications.

I wrote this book in three equal parts. In the first part, I describe the various forms human malaise takes. In the second part, I explain it, provide the why or what is causing us to behave so badly. Based on the explanation in the third part, I provide solutions. It can be a challenge to read, so you have to apply yourself.

Polgar, A.T. (2019). A brief history of how bad behaviour evolved into illness. In R.M. Reynolds (Ed.), ***Miscellaneous Musings*** (pp. 155-175). Retrieved from www.xlibris.com

I wrote this in an effort to inform both professional and lay persons of alternative information about psychiatry and its primary intervention tool, drugs. The intent also was to make it an easy read.

Szasz, T. (1961). ***The myth of mental illness: Foundations of a theory of personal conduct.*** New York, NY: Dell Publishing Co..

One of the first psychiatrists to warn people of the dangers posed by this discipline. A classic that was compulsory reading when I was a student. A practice that should be revisited.

Szasz, T. (1970). ***Ideology and insanity: Essays on the psychiatric dehumanization of man.*** New York, NY: Anchor Books.

The title of this book says it all. The point of it is that Szasz continued to advance his position about the inappropriate medicalization of everyday problems all humans encounter.

Tickle, P. (2004). ***Greed: The seven deadly sins***. New York, NY: Oxford University Press.

One of seven, noted scholars who wrote about the seven deadly sins. Tickle calls greed the mother of all sins and hints at its prevalence to be a function of cognitive developmental stagnation. An easy, informative read.

Whitaker, R. & Cosgrove, L. (2015). ***Psychiatry under the influence***. New York, NY: Palgrave McMillan.

This is a rather easy-to-read history of the emergence of psychiatry as a formidable, global entity. The authors see the problem as attributable to many factors beyond the agenda of individuals or even a single organization.

Yong, E. (2018, June 21). ***A landmark study on the origins of alcoholism.*** The Atlantic. Retrieved from https://www.theatlantic.com/science/archive/2018/06/a-landmark-study-in-the-origins-of-alcoholism/563372/

Reporting on the work of Markus Heilig, this article is one more example of research to justify biological psychiatry. Also a great example of conceptual blurriness, treating alcoholism as if it is a real thing as opposed to addicts who prefer alcohol as long as it is available.

ACKNOWLEDGMENTS

I continue to be grateful and amazed at the unconditional tolerance of Drina, the love of my life. Without question, she supports my tilting at windmills and my stubborn efforts to improve all our lives in spite of many formidable obstacles. In this instance, and in good company, not taking on the discipline of psychiatry, but the historically chronic, global malaise that allowed psychiatry's imperialistic success.

I am grateful for having known Mary (not her real name), whose avoidable, tragic death is the inspiration for this book. She was a wonderful, formidable person, who unfortunately got caught up in a vicious undertow she could not escape. Hopefully, others can learn from her experience and death.

I am grateful for the skillful, tenacious Laura Riggs. She perseveres, in spite of the challenges that is the price for working with me. Not only does she create a beautiful text from what I give her, she also edits and fine tunes, when I lose my way. The scholarly David Angels also had a part in the final editing of the manuscript

I am equally grateful for the continued and most excellent, navigator services of Grant D. Fairley. He is the highly skilled, wise-through-experience pilot who guides our ship to port effortlessly, each and every time. To boot, he is a pleasure to work with.

Last, but by no means least, I am eternally grateful for the principled, scholarly work of others who have, and continue to influence my thinking enormously. Some I reference in this book but there are many others.

ABOUT THE AUTHOR

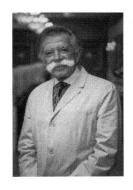

Almost fifty years of curiously pursuing clinical knowledge and skills has brought Alexander T. Polgar Ph.D. to that age and stage in life at which he is even less inclined to tip-toe around the establishment and all that it holds to be sacred.

In this book he dares to dissect the myths created by the establishment's darling psychiatry. True to his form, his approach is to synthesise existing information into a unified evidence based theory. He then makes the information optimally accessible through a story format told in the voice of the protagonist Sally. He does this in pursuit of eradicating conditions that obstruct the cognitive developmental potential with which we are all born. The freedom that this creates, Alex believes, is a prerequisite to addressing with relevant strategies addiction and the maladaptive ways many of us cope with the vagaries of life.

FINDING PURPOSE AND MEANING: SALLY SURVIVES HER BRIEF, NASTY DANCE WITH PSYCHIATRY

This third book of four in a trilogy about substance abuse, delves into the dark realm of how addicts, struggling with abstinence, are inadvertently intoxicated by psychiatrist prescribed drugs when they seek help for problems from which they hid by using. The dangers of dancing with biological psychiatry and their prescribed drugs is extensively explored in this volume. While some pay with their lives for the dance, others like Sally, get off the dance floor to live not only for another day, but an altogether different life. Abstinent, they find purpose and meaning to their life as they start to actualize the gift of innate cognitive developmental potential given to all of us.

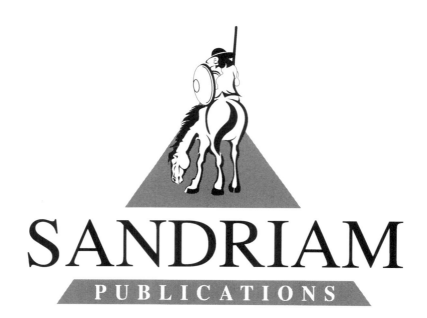

SANDRIAM

PUBLICATIONS

Manufactured by Amazon.ca
Bolton, ON

35576440R00067